Breathe Deep...Now Hold It!

I0173439

*A*dvantage
BOOKS

WHY CHRISTIANS SHOULDN'T PRACTICE YOGA

MICHAEL MUSTO

Breath Deep...Now Hold It by Michael Musto
Copyright © 2023 by Michael Musto
All Rights Reserved.
ISBN: 978-1-59755-726-9

Published by: ADVANTAGE BOOKS™
                     Longwood, Florida, USA
                     www.advbookstore.com

This book and parts thereof may not be reproduced in any form, stored in a retrieval system or transmitted in any form by any means (electronic, mechanical, photocopy, recording or otherwise) without prior written permission of the author, except as provided by United States of America copyright law.

Scriptures marked NKJV are taken from the Holy Bible NEW KING JAMES VERSION®. Copyright© 1982 by Thomas Nelson, Inc. Used by permission. All rights reserved.

Scriptures marked KJV are taken from the Holy Bible KING JAMES VERSION (KJV) which is public domain.

Library of Congress Catalog Number: 2023932297

Editor: nancysabatinicopyedit@gmail.com

First Printing: February 2023
23 24 25 26 27 28   10 9 8 7 6 5 4 3 2 1

TABLE OF CONTENTS

INTRODUCTION

I suspect you looked at the title of this book and felt an urge to at least read the introduction. What was your reason? Did it upset you? Did it make your blood boil with echoes of "That's just wrong" or "I'd like to tell him a thing or two" or something worse running through you head.

Well, you're welcome to read on, but let me warn you it's not going to get any better for you. Remember that a closed mind learns nothing.

However, if you are a Christian who is thinking of practicing Yoga, a Christian already practicing, or someone who wants to hear all sides, then we can make a go of it. I'm not going to tell you what to think or do. I'm just going to tell the story of my journey, after which you can decide on your own.

First, who am I? For the last thirty years I've been a writer and a journalist, working mostly for magazines.

After much thought, I've decided not to use the real names of the people and places mentioned in this book. Not to protect the innocent; there are no innocents. It is best for all concerned that we disregard most names.

Also, much of what we'll discuss has a Sanskrit name or title. Sanskrit is the ancient language of India; sacred scriptures and classical Indian epic poems are written in Sanskrit. To save time and confusion, we'll call them by their role and action, only.

Of course, the two main themes running through this book are: Christianity and Yoga. I'm not a specialist in either one. As a Christian, I am not a pastor, theologian, or an apologetic. When I practiced Yoga, I was not a Guru or a Sage, although I studied and taught Yoga for many years.

However, now I am a Born-Again Christian taking my faith extremely seriously, and have, and continue to study and grow in my relationship with Jesus Christ each passing day.

I guess you can say I've been a seeker all my life, like so many others. This can be a good thing; however, it can also lead you down some strange paths.

As for Yoga, when involved in it, I had the same strong commitment that I do now in my Christian walk. I lived and studied in an Ashram (a hermitage, a community where students and devotees study religious as well as Yogic practices) for two years. After which, I taught Yoga for eight years, while I continued my Yogic studies.

****

So, what is Yoga? The word Yoga is from ancient Sanskrit; it means to yoke or unite. You practice Yoga to earn a union of your individual consciousness with that of the Universal Consciousness. Read that again, and seriously consider what it says - more on this later.

****

Let's do a quick experiment relevant to what we are going to be looking at.

First, physical exercises taught in Yoga may surprise you how easy some of them are, discounting all visions of twisting yourself into a human pretzel.

However, complicated exercises we'll discuss later down the road. This comes in time. Yoga for beginners is really not that difficult.

Important - Read the instruction first because you'll be performing the exercises with your eyes closed.

Sit on a simple dining room chair, back straight, away from the back of the chair, head held high, and feet flat on the floor. Now, grab your knees, pulling gently and slowly pushing your spine forward, as you take in a slow deep breath while moving the chest forward. If you feel any discomfort, stop.

Next, relax the muscles in your arms; slowly pull your spine back till it curves, all the while, slowly exhaling, do this five or six times.

Again, sit up straight. Let your head fall forward, give it no support until your head is hanging and your chin is close to your chest without forcing it. Never force a movement, or you could hurt yourself.

Relax, then, going counter-clock wise, start doing neck-rolls, breathing in as you bring the head back, and exhale as you bring it forward. Don't force it. If you feel any kinks, that snap, crackle, pop sound, go passed them, gently. Do this five or six times, and then stop.

Now do the neck-rolls in the opposite direction. Again, remember the breathing. Do this five or six times, being as gentle as possible, and then stop.

Now hold your head high. Bring you shoulders up, and slowly and gently roll your shoulders backwards. Breathe in when going back and out when coming forward. Do this five or six times, and then stop.

Now roll your shoulders in the opposite direction. Don't forget the breathing.

After five or six times, stop, sit up straight, taking in a long, slow deep breath, and then let it out, slowly.

All breathing is through the nose. Lastly, take in a deep breath, hold it for three seconds, and let it out, slowly.

Relax for a few seconds. Open your eyes.

Congratulations! You've just completed a Yoga session, a simple one, to be sure, but Yoga, nonetheless.

If you performed the exercises correctly, going at a slow and gentle pace, you should be feeling a physical difference, only slight, as it was far from an intense workout.

Still, you should feel a lot looser in you muscles and calmer in your nerves, and a slight increase in blood circulation.

In short, you should feel better than before. You just did something that improved you in some small way.

So, now you're saying, "I just did some simple stretching, where is the harm in that?" I asked those same words when I first started out practicing Yoga, and repeated it for many years after, until, like a snake it bit me and the poison filled me.

The short answer is "Nothing is wrong with it." Stretching and movement is good for you. But there's more to it than that. It's not where you start with Yoga that's wrong, it's where it takes you, and where you end that goes against our Christian Beliefs.

That is one of the biggest dangers of Yoga. At first, it seems innocent and helpful. And it is, at first. In time, it becomes your life, your spiritual path, and the benefits turn into a search for more powers and ungodly things.

The long answer...? This book is the long answer. It is my journal of more than ten years from start to finish.

With a Yoga lifestyle come many disciplines. Some seem strange, some are beneficial. The physical exercises are just a part of the lifestyle. Beneficial or not, it's where it takes you that's important.

Again, the physical exercises play just a small part. And the physical discipline is not necessarily there for your health. The true and finally goal of all Yoga disciplines is spiritual – to connect your individual consciousness with that of the Universal Consciousness and to a reach self-awareness – Enlightenment.

As I stated at the beginning of this introduction, the closed mind learns nothing. So, open your mind, read on, and at the end it's for you to decide.

1 Thessalonians 5:21: Test all things; hold fast what is good. NKJV

Chapter One

Beginnings

Growing up in a small tight-knit community with a loving, and churchgoing family does not insure the child will not wander. I was that wandering child.

Proverbs 22:6: Train up a child in the way he should go, And when he is old he will not depart from it. *KJV*

This Proverb almost implies that a time may come when a child gets off-track. I certainly did.

As a small child, Bible stories intrigued me. Adam and Eve eating the apple, Noah's Ark, Jonah, the baby Moses floating down the Nile in a basket, The Red Sea parting, and afterwards we sang *Yes, Jesus loves me.*

Don't misunderstand, this makes for a great start. Only, there comes a time when we need to start preparing for the world, and at an early age, because the world's call starts early and is very strong.

In time, the luster began to fade. I'd sit with my family in church staring at the stained-glass windows, daydreaming. Whatever preached, I tuned it out. I stopped reading my Bible. I'd lost all interest, and nothing and no one, including my parents were going to bring it back.

After graduating high school, I couldn't wait to be out on my own. And my falling away from the church then didn't compare to how far I would drift in the coming years.

Like so many other young people when they enter the world, scores of them go astray, as I did. The pull of the world is strong and confusing. There's college, peer pressure, music, movies, television, magazines, the media, all of it telling you how wrong you are, and how right you can be.

If you were to ask me at the time if I was a good person, I would have said, "yes". Believing in God, praying when in trouble, helping others, never killing, or stealing, or lying, this makes a good person…right?

Still, my faith was on the backburner. Christianity didn't fit well in my world. There was no appeal and rightfully so; faithless Christianity is nothing more than a boring, soulless, lifeless religion.

Kym was a journalist like me. We weren't the closest of friends, yet our friendship was unique. We were both seekers. Looking high and low for the truth; however, in all the wrong places.

You can tell a seeker by the courses they take in college, the careers they're attracted to, and the lifestyle and friends they keep.

You can also tell a seeker by the books in their home library. Volumes on self-help, astrology, crystals, alternative medicine, spiritualism, witchcraft, UFOs, and the like, and of course no seeker's library would be complete without books on Eastern philosophy and religion.

It's interesting, how Westerners are drawn to all things Eastern, having a soft spot in their hearts for its holy men, unlike Easterners. I found this out firsthand.

I remember when the world-famous Yogi, Iyengar, came to tour America with a series of lectures and classes. Known for founding his own style of Yoga, named after himself, he was a healthy elderly man with long white hair and matching eyebrows as large as eagle's wings, covering most of his forehead.

I was one of the lucky few to attend one of his classes.

It was clear from the start; the man was far advanced in Yoga; however, his teaching-methods upset everyone.

He hollered and basically bullied almost everyone in the class. He left some of the more sensitive students in tears.

That evening, I received an invitation with a few other Yoga teachers to dine with the man who terrorized the entire class throughout the day. They held it at one of the major country clubs, an Indian dinner of all his favorite dishes. The chef outdid himself, and served it with pride.

All through dinner, I couldn't help noticing the man was a fun-loving, mild-mannered gentleman, absolutely different from the tyrant who'd taught the Yoga class only a few hours ago.

I turned to his assistant for an answer.

"That is the way you teach in India," his assistant told me. "I tried to explain to him how self-motivated Americans are; unlike the Indian people that have to be pushed and prodded because they have no interest. You have to be a strong-handed father to such children."

****

"Did you know there's actually an Indian Ashram in this city?" Kym asked over the phone one night, his voice popping with excitement. "And they give Yoga lessons. Not free, mind you, but dirt cheap. They just want to make enough to keep the place open. I've gone to their classes three times. It's great! You've just got to come. They've got classes every night. What night are you free?"

That's how it started, innocent enough. They had classes for beginners, intermediate, and advanced. We attended the beginners' class, of course. Those living at the Ashram taught all the classes, all of them Hindu, some natural born to it, and a few American converts.

Over the next few years, I found this to be very common and widespread. There are many young Americans seeking for something to believe in. Some never received an ounce of religious training in their youth, others strayed from what they were raised on.

For them it was a break into something different, a different life with a new name, new dress, new diet, and a whole new lifestyle.

The Ashram was in a seedy part of town. One hundred years earlier it was the wealthiest part of town, which accounted for so many large mansions spotted throughout the area. Now being one of the poorer parts of the city, these mansions went for a song. Many entrepreneurs bought them and turned them into apartment buildings. However, this one particular mansion found rebirth as a Yoga Ashram.

My first impressions were mixed; understandably, after all, it was a different culture.

It was a four-story building, housing six devotees, all of them Yoga teachers. The rooms were large and open, with little to no furniture. The main room, which must have been a ballroom at one time in the past, they now used for Yoga classes. It was a completely empty room, save for carpets fully covering the floor, and a large gong, on which a mallet hung. The walls were solid white with framed paintings and old black and white photos of well-known ancient and once passed Gurus – teachers of Yoga. In time to come, I would learn all their names and then some.

The place was clean with an air of tranquility abounding. The teachers were friendly, as were my fellow students. As well, each of the teachers were...how should I put this...charismatic with a manner of serenity and inner wisdom. At least that was my impression, at the time.

Yoga has many strange practices and philosophies, most of which beginners never hear, and only few of the intermediates. These mysteries are for the serious advanced students. We'll look at these later.

However, I would like to say something to their credit. Despite all this, Yoga is not a cult. The dedication and the addiction some people have for Yoga makes it feel like one, at times. These people believe in what they are doing; they see it as helping the human race. If it's not for you, then so be it. Nothing and no one are making you stay. Although, for some, leaving is near impossible.

My first class went great. It was not too difficult, no impossible poses; nothing considered particularly strange, just stretching, heavy breathing, and relaxing. When it was over, I felt good, no more so than a trip to the gym or water aerobics, but it was more in tune with my head during that time in my life.

I left with full intent on returning. In fact, I signed and paid in advance for three more months of classes, twice each week. I didn't miss one.

****

The weeks flew by, each class got easier. They alternated the teachers, and in time we got to know all of them, as well as getting to know the other students. All nice people, they were.

It's a true fact; you are the company you keep. There was a time I would have questioned some of what I heard and saw, but being around like minds made it all commonplace. In many ways, we fed off one another, and urged each other on. We introduced our beliefs to one another, as if pushing an agenda, till we were all fully indoctrinated with all the New Age culture had to offer.

A bond also formed with the teachers. Everyone had their favorites; however, we liked each for different reasons. Although, there was something common about each of them, they gave the impression they knew something we didn't, something we lacked, something we needed if we were ever to live a happy and fruitful life. There needed to be a balance of mind, body, and spirit. And the power needed to succeed was in us, not outside us. No God could help us, for we are just as powerful, if only we could tap into that power. Somewhere along the line, we forgot our greatness, our true and higher self, and Yoga was the path to regain it.

It all became very social, both in and out of class. Sometimes, there were dinners with the teachers after class. It was all extremely interesting, both the food, which was always vegan, and the conversation, which was always New Age in drift. There were trips together to vegan restaurants, hikes through parks and around lakes. It all seemed totally innocent.

Then there were the trips to Hindu Temples. By now, nothing seemed odd or questionable. After all, god is god. Even though some don't know it or willing to see and admit it, all seek and worship the same god. Right…?

Of course, many students came and went. It was the serious ones that continued - hungry for more, to continue up the never ending ladder to enlightenment. The next rung was coming, and I was ready.

Chapter Two

Tip of the Iceberg

Intermediate classes were far more intense. The exercises were more of a challenge, an extreme workout.

Save for the physical, other aspects came into play, and the list was long. Meditation, Chanting and Breathing exercises became a regular part of the class.

The other part that became prevalent was it was now clearly becoming a spiritual quest.

It was then that the truths about Yoga came into light. This is the part few people know, and what is sure to anger some that hear me speak it.

There are many facets to practicing Yoga; however, for now, we are just looking at the physical exercises. The truth is, these exercises are useful to one's health; no question, other than that, they are not the main goal. I repeat: Good health, though highlighted and sought after, is not the goal of Yoga.

The main reason is to prepare the body to raise the life-power that lies nearly idle deep within us. This rising makes us more powerful and allows us to connect with the Universal Consciousness, god, enlightenment, or what have you.

This power goes by many names. In the orient, mostly in the martial arts, they call it Qi, also Ki, or Ch'i (pronounced Chee). Translation: vital force or simply – energy. In India it is called the Kundalini, the life force.

Without the correct training, raising the Kundalini can be dangerous. That is why the emphasis on the physical. This Kundalini, this powerful life force, rushing up the unprepared spine can leave a person damaged, to say the least.

They told me many of the so-called Christian saints raised their Kundalini at great risk to themselves, Saint Francis of Assisi for one.

It surprised me to learn the Bible refers to all Believers as Saints and Children of God.

Ephesians 2:19: Now therefore ye are no more strangers and foreigners, but fellow citizens with the saints, and of the household of God... KJV

John 1:12: But as many as received Him, to them He gave the right to become children of God, to those who believe in His name... NKJV

It's said the Kundalini, this life force, lies dormant at the base of the spine. The purpose of Yoga is to prepare the body to channel this force up the spine to the top of the head; from there it will connect with the infinite.

In short, even if you are innocently practicing Yoga for your health, you are playing with forces you are not even aware of and do not understand. And in that vulnerable state you are leaving yourself open for all and every force, including demonic, no different from the way drugs open such portholes.

Lately, even many Christian churches offer courses in Yoga, saying they don't do the religionist part of the practice; they only do the physical exercises. Again, they're misinformed and playing with unknown forces. There is no nonreligious part to Yoga. For a Christian, there is no innocent side to Yoga.

That's like drinking four Screwdrivers and saying you won't get drunk because you're only going to drink the orange juice and spit out the vodka. It can't be done. They can not be separated.

The practice of Yoga, the exercises, the breathing, the mediations, the diet, not only prepares the body, but also stimulates and coaxes the Kundalini up the spine.

The rise of the Kundalini may take years or a minute, and everything in between, maybe even more than one lifetime, so they claim. It all depends on the person's practice and Karma, which we will discuss later.

As the Kundalini rises in the spine it passes through seven Chakras along the way, stimulating each as it passes through.

The word "Chakra" in ancient Sanskrit means "Wheel". Chakras are points in the body, spinning disks of energy that serve the body. They say there are many more; however, the seven main Chakras are the main focus. In most people these terminals of energy are sluggish or even blocked to a stand still. They must remain open and in good working order.

The seven Chakras are thus:

1.   Root Chakra –at the base of the spine, the tailbone area. This is where we harbor our physical and emotional being.

2.   Sacral Chakra – it's slightly under the bellybutton. Here is our creativity, pleasure, and sexuality.

3.   Solar Plexus Chakra – found in the stomach area. Here we find our sense of worth and confidence.

4.   Heart Chakra – found at the center of the chest. This is the center of love and compassion.

5.   Throat Chakra – found at the throat. This Chakra affects how we communicate with others and the world around us.

6.   Third Eye Chakra – found at the forehead, between the eyes. Here we house our imagination and intuition.

7.   Crown Chakra – found at the top of the head. We find here our awareness, our intelligence. Here we connect with the infinite – Enlightenment.

As the Kundalini life force travels up the spine, it connects with these Chakras. It stimulates them and opens them. In turn, the qualities controlled by the Chakra become heightened, more powerful, to the point of being Superhuman, mentally, physically, and spiritually.

****

This was only the tip of the iceberg. There was much more to come. But it was exciting and hopeful. How could anyone think poorly of Yoga? After all, look at what it had to offer, only good things.

Yoga offered better health, for one. Who doesn't want better health? But there was so much more. I could become a calmer and more stable person with a creative mind, a more compassionate soul, loving and loved by others. The promise was like a carrot dangling from a string in front of me, and I was hungry.

It all made so much sense. This is a world of action and reaction, a world of works. You do this, which makes that happens. And you have the power to make it so. You don't need anyone or anything, just yourself. You don't even need God. In fact, maybe, just maybe, we might all be gods.

Chapter Three

The Big Move

As pointed out before, years ago the building that became the Ashram was once a rich family's mansion. As an Ashram, it was a catacomb of rooms. The kitchen and dining area were huge, with a large refrigerator that devotees shared, each getting an assigned area.

As well, the once ballroom where young debutants and their beaus danced the night away was overly large with a high ceiling from which hung a great chandelier, and a deep well of a fireplace at one wall. It was now the room where they held classes with people sitting cross-legged on the floor.

All the other rooms they'd converted into bedrooms, one for each devotee to live in and decorate as their own. They were responsible for the furnishings and cleanness of their room. Bathrooms, on every floor, were down the hall, with one large bathroom on the main floor for the students.

One night at the end of our intermediate class, they announced that one of the devotees would be leaving, meaning one of the bedrooms would be vacant, and would anyone consider moving in.

I don't think anyone in the class gave it a second thought, including me. After all, I had a good life. After a day's work, I'd come home to my stylish apartment, do what I wanted, eat what I wanted, and live the way I wanted. It was my own little world, and I didn't have to share. Sure, the rent at the Ashram was far less than what I was paying; and the person that moved in would eventually become a Yoga teacher. This meant extra money. But that was not enough incentive.

Why would anyone want to live in an Ashram? Living with other people in what one can only describe as a commune, and that went out with the hippies.

However, for the next week I couldn't stop thinking of the offer. Every time I weighted the choices, it didn't add up. Still, there was an attraction that drew me in. Finally, against my better judgment, I decided to go for it.

Of course, all the residents had to approve of me, first; which they did. And there were house rules that needed following, or they'd ask you to leave. They voted me in with flying colors.

I paid my first month's rent. That was a good feeling. It was a third of what I normally paid each month. They showed me my portion of the refrigerator, and parking space in the back. Before moving in, I gave away rooms of furniture. I only had the one room, now.

Honestly, the house rules were understandable for what it was. Your room was your room, and you needed to take care of it, as well as help keep the building clean. We took turns cleaning the bathrooms and the kitchen.

I must admit, everyone tried to have at least a decent relationship with the others. There was a weekly meeting of the residents; it was all very civilized. In all the time I lived there, I never heard an uncivil word spoken.

All shared the kitchen; as well as utensils, so always clean up after use. They also assigned sections of the cupboards.

It was important to live as a vegan, if not at least a vegetarian. They'd tolerate butter and other dairy products, although when using such ingredients we would not use the house utensils. Always leave the kitchen the way you found it, the bathrooms as well. Under the Ashram laws you had to be a clean freak, which was good.

Of course, there was no way of knowing what goes on in your room behind closed doors, but house rules were clear: no sexual encounters with other devotees or guests from the outside world.

Still, they allowed guests of the opposite sex in your room, until ten o'clock. You were on your honor there'd be no hanky-panky. You could go to someone else's house and do what you wanted; however, that left you feeling guilty, and rightfully so.

As for me, it was a time in my life I held no interest for such behavior, and now thinking about it, again, it was a good thing.

With my living at the Ashram came many perks besides low-rent, companionship, we always had one another's backs, and lived in a serene atmosphere. No one was overly loud; in fact, no one was overly anything, mostly keeping to themselves. There was a extensive library at my deposal. The books were on Yoga, Gurus, Eastern Religion, and many New Age topics. Some of the books were commonplace found in any New Age bookstore; some were not only rare, but were no longer in print. It was a Yoga devotee's candy store.

I was always welcome at all the Hindu Temples within one hundred miles, I went only on special occasions, and in time it no longer felt uncomfortable, and became second nature to me. After all, all of us worship the same god…don't we? It's just the way we worship him or her that separates us…right?

Many of the Ashrams across this country are somewhat, if not completely, connected with one another; they are at the least willing to help other Ashrams.

Often, well-known Yoga Teachers, Swamis, and Gurus, from all over the world, especially India, come to this country to teach, lecture, sell books, and what have you. Sometimes, even musicians on tour from India would stay over. They relied on the network of Ashrams for lodging and transport.

It was commonplace to receive a phone call to pick up a famous guest and their entourage at the airport. We'd fix a room for them, and cook a scrumptious supper in their honor.

We considered ourselves blessed to have such elite guests stay at our Ashram. In exchange for our hospitality, we received the right to sit at the master's feet, and, as they say, hear it straight from the horse's mouth.

The next day we'd drive them to their destination, a lecture or a book signing. Then that night, again, bring them back to the Ashram for another wonderful meal and time at the foot of the master. The next morning, we drove them to the airport, and they'd fly out to the next Ashram, wherever that may be.

To be honest, thinking back now, I enjoyed the musicians the most. Their visits were much more pleasurable.

Of all these perks, the top perk was the Yoga classes.

As a devotee and resident of the Ashram, I could attend every class I wanted for free, and attend I most defiantly did.

There were as many as a dozen classes, beginners, intermediate, and advanced, each week, and I felt determined to be at as many as possible.

In only a few short months, the others living and teaching at the Ashram approached me to teach Yoga classes, for beginners only, of course. I even became a certified teacher.

I felt honored. Now, I felt more motivated than ever.

Chapter Four

Meditation

Usually, beginner Yoga classes consist of nothing more than exercises with simple controlled breathing. The most you can expect is calm music, and not much else.

Seeing how most people never go beyond the beginner phrase, it surprises them if anyone criticizes Yoga. After all, what's so wrong about stretching to soft music while you breathe deeply?

It isn't until you advance to intermediate are other issues brought in.

The next and one of the most prevalent additions is the practice of mediation.

However, before we can go any further we need to have a working understanding of what we mean by "Meditation" in this case.

There's a big difference from what the Western world considers Meditation, compared to the Eastern world.

Meditation in the West is nothing more than deep thinking, focusing and or reflecting on the thought within one's mind.

Eastern or Yoga Meditation is a horse of a different color. Yes, it is focusing on the mind; yet, it's mostly done silently in the mind with aids, such as chanting, use of a mantra, specific breathing, all for religious and spiritual advancement.

The Westerner meditates on something; the Easterner tries to empty the mind, to be thoughtless.

The intent and outcome are also quite different. In the West we meditate to get a better understanding of what we are meditating on. Eastern Meditation is done for a varied amount of reasons, which we'll discuss along the way. But, first, let's look at the basics.

Sit cross-legged on the floor, preferably on a soft surface such as a carpet or a rug. Keep the spine straight, but remain relaxed and comfortable. Breathe normally through your nose; however, make the breaths long and slow. Once you are comfortable, relax deeply, close your eyes and try to clear you mind.

Of course, removing thought from the mind is not easy, especially for beginners.

Depending on the teacher, the style of Yoga you are studying, and the particular meditation you are practicing, Mantras can be whispered within or spoken aloud . To start off, we will look at the inner Mantra.

Silently in your mind, repeat the Mantra given to you. A Mantra is a sound, word, or short phrase spoken in ancient Sanskrit. The vibrations of these sounds affect the mind, slowing it down, and eventually, with practice, emptying it.

Just keep repeating the Mantra, trying to remove all thoughts. If a thought appears in you mind, don't get upset or discouraged, reset your mind and return to repeating the Mantra.

It may seem difficult or even impossible the first few times you try this; however, in time with practice, it gets easier, and you can increase the time of the meditation. Beginners start at five to ten minutes, increasing over time in small increments.

An hour is commonly the goal. However, there are well-known Yogis who they say can do this practice for days.

Even for the beginner, some results are immediate. You should feel calmer at the finish than when you started.

Again, you may ask "Calmer? And what's wrong with that?" Nothing, of course; however, again, there's more here than meets the eye.

Interestingly, scientists have studied this phenomenon only to find the same results can be achieved by sitting calmly and using any word you like in place of a so called holy Mantra. It's even accomplished by using random names from the phonebook.

As I said, the example of meditation just given is just your common everyday style. There are as many types of meditations as there are teachers, with variations to boot.

Relaxation is just a by-product of Mediation. The reasons to practice are many, the first being able to maneuver the Kundalini (the life energy) up the spine, activating the Chakras, and eventually connecting with the infinite.

The reasons to meditate reads like the ultimate human wish list. There are meditations to promote prosperity, good health, mental clarity, pregnancy, ward off diseases, be able to see the future, see visions, hear voices, time-travel, astral projection(leave your body), answer prayers, gain wisdom, and thousands of other expected outcomes.

Meditation can include specific breathing, and chants, which we'll look at in the next few chapters.

As for the Mantras, an important part of many meditations, it creates a resonance that affects the body and sprit.

To the ear not trained in Sanskrit, they sound like beautiful, nonsensical, foreign words, and sometimes that's all they are.

However, some are phrases or names of deities repeated over and over, as it is with chanting. On the other hand, what a Hindu considers a deity, a Christian will declare an evil spirit or demon.

As mentioned before, some well-intentioned Christians claim to practice a form of Meditation that is in line with Christianity: such as repeating the names of God or phrases from the Bible. It is still mindless repetition, which the Bible warns us to avoid.

Matthew 6:7: But when ye pray, use not vain repetition, as the heathens do: for they think they shall be heard for their much speaking. KJV

Now, let's take a look into the philosophy behind Meditation, which to the student with little or no understanding of Christianity will find logical and nothing more than good clear thinking.

The Universal Mind is perfect, all knowing and without flaw, whereas, the mind of the individual is imperfect and limited.

The thoughts in the mind of the individual, being imperfect and limited, only cause havoc and chaos, which steers us away from our true goal.

When we abandon our thoughts, empty our mind, the Universal Mind takes charge. Being perfect and unlimited, it will guide us to our goal, and in time, connect with the individual mind...better known as enlightenment.

****

The Christian doesn't empty the mind; they fill it with the word of God.

The Christian doesn't focus so much on the self; Jesus is our main focus.

The Christian finds their calmness by resting in the Lord

The Christian doesn't look to control; God is in control.

The Christian doesn't try to escape life; they seek guidance from the Holy Spirit.

James 1:17: Every good gift and every perfect gift is from above, and cometh down from the Father of lights, with whom is no variableness, neither shadow of turning. KJV

Chapter Five

Chanting

There are as many differences as there are likenesses between Mantras and Chanting. Now, we're not talking about Georgian Chants or Psalms. This is an entirely different animal.

True, usually the chant will be musical in nature, but it is in no way a song. It can stand alone, or used as a Mantra.

It's believed sounding words in a particular order, causes a vibration that affects the Yogi in the same way a Mantra does.

You can chant during an exercise or during a meditation, or alone as the mediation.

Chanting in Yoga is a group of Sanskrit words, repeated silently in the mind, whispered, said aloud, or, on rare occasions, shouted. Often, a chant may have a coinciding breathing technique, as well as specific finger positions, which we'll discuss later in another chapter.

Again, as with a Mantra we have repetition of words, which the Bible warns against.

Like the Mantras in meditation, a chant will decrease stress, anxiety, depression, and improve you mood and increase your focus. And as with Mantras, it has been scientifically proven that you can get the same results from just sitting, relaxing, and pondering. Many Christians claim that deep contemplation on a Bible passage gives them the same outcome.

Besides acting as a Mantra, the reasons for Chanting are many, mostly personal gain, such as happiness, strength, money, success, health. However, you can chant for things like compassion and empathy.

I've even met some Yogis that do a chant of protection before they enter a car, or a boat, a plane, or any form of travel. I always found it amusing to see them chant not only when getting into the vehicle, but if they stopped, get out for some reason, and then returned, they'd chant, again. It would seem the power of the chant didn't last the day, and would need another chant every time you stop and go.

So, in a sense, Chanting is an incantation. An incantation is a group of words said as a magic spell or charm.

Ezekiel 13:20: Therefore thus says the Lord GOD: "Behold, I am against your magic charms by which you hunt souls there like birds. I will tear them from your arms, and let the souls go, the souls you hunt like birds. NKJV

As with the Mantras, the Sanskrit words often invoke the many names of gods, Shiva, Buddha, Vishnu, and many more. Occasionally, the word "god" is chanted. Of course, it is not specific which god we're talking about. Some of the more well-known chants are;

- Om Mani Padme Hum = Hail to the jewel in the lotus (referring to the Buddha)

- Om Namah Shivaya = I bow to Shiva

- Om Gum Ganapatayei Namah = I bow to Ganesh the elephant faced deity

This is only the tip of the iceberg. There are thousands of chants. But, you catch my drift.

Isaiah 45:5: I am the Lord thy God, and there is none else, there is no God beside me... KJV

Here we read Isaiah reintegrating the first of the Ten Commandments. Interesting, that God put it first; it must be very important, don't you think?

Chapter Six

Mudras

Mudra, an ancient Sanskrit word, means gesture or attitude. It can also mean pose. Though never mentioned at classes for beginners and seldom at classes for intermediates, Mudras play an important part of advanced Yoga studies.

The hand and finger positioning is important, aiding on multiple levels such as spiritual, emotional, and the physic plane. The correct Mudras give support to the energy flow helping the individual connect with the Universe or Cosmos.

Many Yogis, including Buddhists and Hindus and many more, consider Mudras as sacred.

There are hundreds of Mudra combinations. Each Mudra, hand and finger position affects the mind and body, helping clear energy pathways, creating a straight course for the Kundalini to rise.

You can perform the Mudras not only during physical exercises. They're often performed during meditations and breathing exercises.

Although hand and finger gestures are the most common, other body parts can come into play, the throat, eyes, stomach, diaphragm, just to name a few. They call these Bandah, which means "Lock". You tighten or lock the muscles involved and then relax or release, having an affect on the practitioner.

Some of the more well-known Mudras are:

- Gyan Mudra – The tip of the thumb and the index finger touch, the other fingers extended, and the palm facing upwards. The most commonly used in meditation, it's believed to calm the mind.

- Dhyana Mudra – Right hand rests on top of the left, palms up, creating a cup-like formation, thumbs touching. This famous Mudra was a favorite of the Buddha.

- Anjali Mudra – Palms together, held at the chest, fingers pointing upward, often called the "Prayer Pose."

- Bhu Mudra – Curl fingers and thumbs into the palms, point to or touch the ground. This helps you connect with the earth – your Mother Earth.

Placing the hands and fingers in a pose is only one method. Movement can be part of the Mudra, different fingertips touch one and then another. Also, you might touch the ringlets of the fingers, each movement creating a different effect.

Often when doing these movements, there are Chants that go with the movements, one word or syllable of the chant with each movement.

The next time you see a painting or statue of the Buddha or any Eastern deities, take notice of the hand and finger positions. They will always be performing one of the Mudras.

As well, notice the hands on traditional Indian dancers, their hands will be in a Mudra.

Once again, we find the Yogi caught amid mindless repetition. Not just in thought and word, but in movements, always relying on their own works to carry out what only God can do.

Proverbs 3:5-6: Trust in the LORD with all your heart, and lean not on your own understanding; in all your ways acknowledge Him, and He shall direct your paths. NKJV

Chapter Seven

Breathing

I can imagine right now you're wondering what can be wrong with breathing. Every living thing on this earth breathes. What is wrong with breathing?

Of course, we're talking about controlled breathing, which is a part of all our lives. Everyone experiences and uses this.

We use controlled breathing when we swim, snorkel, exercise, dance, snap photos, shoot a gun, and hundred of other physical activities.

And again, we're talking about something other than our everyday experiences. Yoga looks at breathing as redirecting energy to get a desired result.

Each of us can fundamentally understand this. We practiced a form of this from when we were young until now. All of us remember when as a child we went running to our mothers with tears in our eyes, upset about something. What was her first advice? "Relax, take a deep breath and calm down." And it worked, as soon as our breath was under control; we were able to explain our predicament.

The ancient Yogis introduced this practice with a simple example, it goes like this:

Wherever you travel in India, you will see the mighty elephant, one of the largest and strongest animals, restless, stubborn and defiant. Yet, with nothing more than a short thin stick, the herdsman will make the animal go where he wants it to go and do what he commands.

In Yoga, it is the same. The human mind is strong, restless, stubborn and defiant. Yet, with the control of the breath, the mind will follow and be submissive.

As you may guess, this is only the introduction. There are many styles of controlled breathing, some very intense.

The most common breathing exercise for beginners they call Three-Part Breathing. It goes like this:

<u>Part One</u> – Inhale through your nose, allowing your belly to expand. Then exhale through the nose, tightening your stomach muscles, and drawing your bellybutton toward the spine, forcing as much air out of the lungs as possible.

Part Two – This part is similar to the first, only now the rib cage comes into play, expanding the rib cage on the inhale. On the exhale, squeeze the air out of you rib cage and belly until all air is gone.

Part Three – The same breathing exercise with the upper chest filled as well. Again, exhale fully.

Other common practices are sticking your tongue out, rolling the edges of your tongue to create a funnel. Breathing in through this funnel helps to cool the body.

Or inhale and then hum like a bee as you exhale. The humming causes a resonating vibration in the head and heart. Heightened awareness, mentally, emotionally, and spiritually are the benefits.

You might alternate nostrils by pressing one of the nostrils closed with your index finger, do this as you focus on a Chakra while repeating a Mantra.

Time your inhales and exhales by counting silently.

These are just a few exercises, all of them believed to improve health and further the Yogi's spiritual development, even burning off bad Karma (infractions, or sins, collected in this life and in past lives).

Because of the power dealt with in this exercise, Yogis advise that practitioners go slowly in their studies, and never do more than one breathing exercise during each session.

Breathing exercises can be part of an exercise, a meditation, a chant, or simply stand on its own.

Techniques vary. For instance, breathing in the nose, out the mouth, or visa versa. You may close off one nostril with your finger and breathe through the other or you can alternate nostrils. Long slow breaths, quick short breaths, the combinations are endless, each affecting the nervous system.

Control of the diaphragm is also important. Holding the breath and let it out or holding the breath out and then inhaling. Different time gaps, both in and out, are very common.

One of the most popular breathing exercises they call *Breath of Fire*, easy to learn and do and considered very powerful.

In a sense, you can describe it as huffing. Always through the nose, the mouth remains closed. Breath of Fire is quick-paced, rhythmic, and continuous. Both the inhale and the exhale are equal having no pause between the breaths; as well, the inhale and exhale are never completed. You never take in a full breath or let it out fully. It's done fast – two to three cycles per second. The belly muscles and solar plexus come into play, enhancing the force behind the cycle.

It's suggested the novice start off doing this exercise for a short time, and building slowly to longer and longer periods of practice. I have known some practitioners working up to hours.

They also warn that pregnant women or women on their menstrual cycle should avoid the practice. You should also avoid it if you have high blood pressure, heart disease, or are prone to vertigo or seizures.

They claim many benefits of Breath of Fire, everything from releasing toxins, strengthening the nervous system, better focus, stronger immune system, preventing diseases and much more.

I'm sure by now you're thinking; this sounds a lot like hyperventilating. Yogis say it is something different, and that if you're hyperventilating, you are doing it wrong. Again, if it looks like a duck…

The likenesses are obvious, such as light-headedness, tinkling, especially in the hands, the feet, and the face, dizziness, feeling giddy, and even sometimes going unconscious.

It reminds me so much of when I was a little kid I used to spin around in place and then abruptly stopping, only for the world to keep spinning, and then I'd fall to the floor, laughing.

1 Corinthians 13:11: When I was a child, I spake as a child; I understood as a child, I thought as a child: but when I became a man, I put away childish things. *KJV*

Chapter Eight

Philosophy

Like the ancient Greeks, Plato, Aristotle and Socrates, Yoga Philosophy concerns itself with the individual's mental and physical health, their happiness, and their place in society. Yet, unlike the ancient Greek philosophers, Yoga Philosophy is concerned more with the spiritual and the individual's place in the universe.

The great and the small in the Yoga world, when asked, insist that Yoga is not a religion. In fact, they uphold that a student can continue with their religious beliefs no matter how involved they are in Yoga. This is a contradiction since many of the practices conflict with many religious views, especially Christianity.

Is Yoga a religious? No it isn't. Not in the traditional sense. However, the emphasis on spirituality would make you think otherwise.

As open-minded as it all may seem, I've never met an advancing student that didn't eventually put aside their previous religious beliefs to further their Yoga practice.

Understandably, everyone wants acceptance from their peers. No one wants to be an outsider. In time, the long list of common beliefs in Yoga, the devotees totally accept.

Even something as innocent as vegetarianism has a dark side in Yoga. It's not so much the belief that eating meat will hinder your performance, as do many other foods, such as alcohol and drugs and even certain foods such as vinegar and processed foods, the problem lies with Reincarnation and Karma.

In Yoga, they believe that every creature has a soul, and that the soul lives, dies, and then is reborn. Your conduct and progress in this life decides what life will be your next. Live a good life; earn a good or maybe an even better one. Live a bad life, well...

You may be a human in this life, and then a cow in the next. So, killing a cow or even swatting a fly is initially murder.

There are some Yogis that wear face coverings in fear of inhaling insects, or avoid riding in a boat because the motion of the boat may kill microbes in the water. All souls are the same, all are equal. Believing this offers only one conclusion. We are not created in the image of God.

I've also met some Yogis who are not only vegetarian or vegan, but will not eat root plants (potatoes, carrots, and such) in dread of killing the plant.

Genesis 1:27: So God created man in His own image; in the image of God He created him; male and female He created them.: NKJV

Ephesians 2:8-9: For by grace are ye saved through faith; and that not of yourselves: it is the gift of God: Not of works, lest any man should boast. KJV

The Yogi treasures accumulating knowledge and wisdom. The more knowledge and wisdom the more you can advance. They also believe these memories are never really forgotten, but embedded somewhere within us throughout our lives and any other lives that may follow.

Yoga is a works based journey; although, they wouldn't call the final destination salvation. You hear words like enlightenment, nirvana, connecting with the universal mind or spirit or force. Unlike the salvation instantly offered from God through Jesus Christ, it is a difficult lifelong expedition; perhaps, even multiple, perhaps, thousands of lifetimes, inhabiting many forms, human, animal, insect, and vegetable. While some even believe you can reincarnate as a rock or stone.

Many say we are only trying to remember what we've forgotten. In ancient times, millenniums ago, we were once perfect, a god. Yoga gradually returns this memory back to us.

Although, I do find it strange that if we were once perfect, that is gods, how is it we forgot? It would seem we were not so perfect to start off with.

Perfection cannot become imperfect, or it was never really perfect. And no amount of work can make imperfection turn perfect, even in a million lifetimes. None of us was ever perfect and will never be perfect, not in this life.

Only one person that ever lived was perfect. The only power that can transform an imperfect being is the power of Almighty God.

2 Corinthians 5:21: For He made Him who knew no sin to be sin for us, that we might become the righteousness of God in Him. NKJV

Another prevalent belief in Yoga is Pantheism. It's the belief the world is either indistinguishable to God, or an expression of God's nature. It comes from 'pan' meaning all, and 'theism', which means belief in God. According to pantheism, God is everything and everything is God, you, me, the animals, the rocks and stones, it's all God.

This takes away from the glory that is God. He is the creator not the creation.

In the words of a 20th century philosopher: "For thousands of years, humanity has prayed, fasted, meditated, and still he remains the same."

It is the first lie Satan told the human race.

Genesis 3:5: For God knows that in the day you eat of it your eyes will be opened and you will be like God, knowing good and evil. NKJV

Satan said this long ago; and he's still saying it.

Romans 3:10: As it is written, There is none righteous, no, not one… KJV

Yoga Philosophy believes all people are good; however, past lives and Karma have buried it. We work like a digger with a shovel on the beach, forever trying to overtake the sands of our Karma to the treasure.

Chapter Nine

Reincarnation and Karma

Although I've mentioned Reincarnation in past chapters, we have barely scratched the surface, especially, when it concerns and connects with *Karma*.

Karma is action, deeds, thoughts, or feelings causing an effect to the spirit (the true self) of the devotee. It is also the cause and effect on the physical and spiritual realm. These actions can be good, bad, or neutral. Either way, they become part of the devotee, of their makeup, attached to them, for better or worse. It can be a blessing or a curse.

The good Karma needs increasing and the bad Karma paid for, expelled. This you do, of course, by works, be it action, deeds, thoughts, or feelings. Oddly enough, there are some exercises, meditation, and chants believed to help burn away bad Karma.

They claim that as we go from life to life, we gather or erase both bad Karma and sometimes even good Karma. It's like a scorecard. Only, it will never turn out even. All human beings are flawed and sinful. Reborn as a human with flaws, we cannot become flawless. Without a savior we're doomed to fail, be it for one lifetime or a thousand.

Hebrew 9:27: And as it is appointed for men to die once, but after this the judgment… KJV

If you follow the idea of Reincarnation, its ins and outs, and ups and downs, in time, you can have only one conclusion, and that is the Theory of Evolution.

Anything moving forward has to have a back-there, a beginning. Without God and the Bible, it all makes perfect sense; you can check all the boxes. You were once someone else, and perhaps even an animal, possibly an ameba that crawled out of the slime billions of years ago. It's all a matter of chance and we are all cosmic goo.

I find it interesting that evolutionists believe we were once single-cell creatures, splitting in two for procreation. But isn't the theory based on survival of the fittest?

So, we were once a single-cell, self-contained creature, and now we need another to procreate. Isn't that taking a step in the wrong direction?

Without a Biblical understanding of how things work, the premise of Reincarnation and Karma answers many deep and mystical questions that plagued the human race since the beginning of thought itself.

For instance, everyone's favorite: "Why do bad things happen to good people?"

With Reincarnation and Karma the answer is simple and as clear as the nose on your face.

Through many lifetimes, you have been gathering good and bad Karma. If something bad happens to you in this life, it is because you have to make amends for the wrongs you have done in a past life. It is the same with good fortune. It's all because of your past good works.

When a child dies, or someone suffers, there's no reason for alarm, question, or pity. They're only getting what they deserve. It can actually be a good thing. After all, think of all the bad Karma burning away, no longer carried to the next life.

Romans 5:12: Wherefore, as by one man sin entered into the world, and death by sin; and so death passed upon all men, for that all have sinned: KJV

There is no written law in many of the Yogic beliefs. You can take it or leave it; however, most take it. There are many Yogis that don't believe in Reincarnation, or Karma, or even God.

One of the saddest facets of Reincarnation is it allots time to the Yogi. If you don't get it done today, don't worry, there's always tomorrow and tomorrow and...

I once heard an Indian philosopher, when asked about Reincarnation say, "If you believe in it, aren't you bound to break away from rebirth? What are you doing to escape from this wheel of rebirths?"

Another thing I found disturbing about the Yoga community (not all, but most) is their feelings on abortion.

These people who refuse to eat meat and by-products from animals, people that go out of their way not to hurt a fly, but think nothing of killing a child in the womb. When asked about this, you hear many of the usual explanations we hear from the secular world.

Karma being the payback for your past actions, abortion is just another outcome of those actions. Of course, there are some who don't believe the child is anything other than a growth. Still, there are many who believe it is nothing other than settlement on past debts.

Sadly, I even found many whose religion claims the soul enters the body on the 120th day of pregnancy. How they came up with this time frame, I never learned, and when asked all they did was shrug their shoulders. They don't announce the pregnancy to family and friends, because there is no child before the 120-day mark. Meaning they believe at some point it is a human being. Still, despite this doctrine, they see no reason to speak against prolife, vote against prolife, or have an abortion.

Jeremiah 1:5: Before I formed thee in the belly I knew thee; and before thou camest forth out of the womb I sanctified thee, and I ordained thee a prophet unto the nations. *KJV*

Psalm 139:14: I will praise thee; for I am fearfully and wonderfully made: marvelous are thy works; and that my soul knoweth right well. KJV

Chapter Ten

Life in an Ashram

As you can imagine, living in an Ashram was unique; especially, in contrast to my everyday life. I was leading a double-life, dressed in my everyday street clothes, driving to the office, working my job as always. Yet, I returned each evening to the life of a Yogi.

Ashram life was a combination of college dorm, hippie commune, and Tibetan monastery. For what it was, it was a good experience. Those that lived there were considerate, clean, and reliable.

Some of the devotees worked jobs away from the Ashram, just like I did. However, many remained, teaching Yoga classes throughout the day. We were all financially compensated for the classes we taught. It was slight, still, a great perk.

Every evening, I would teach a class; at first only beginners, in time intermediate, and eventually advance classes, even on weekends.

It was not required, only an invitation, they invited me to attend ceremonies at the Hindu Temple. At first it seemed strange; but, like everything, if you do it often enough it becomes second nature.

It was like living in a bubble. The outside world became a stage-play and I had a bit part to play. My entire life became Yoga. The people around me thought the same; all of us, justifying one another's lives.

****

Over the years, my practice became more expert, and my knowledge of Yoga increased. With it came another distraction in my life.

First, let me say that Yoga didn't cause this distraction directly, that is; but the relationships between students and teachers, as well as Gurus and devotees intensified.

As I stated before, they claim Yoga is not a religion; yet, it comes across as one. And many people involved in Yoga treated it as if it were. As an experienced Yoga teacher, I wasn't only treated well and looked up to as a leader, but also their source for answers – physical, mental, and spiritual.

Students will come to their Yoga teachers with all sorts of ailments, before even consulting a doctor. The teacher regurgitates what they've learned, which they believe to be the truth. Thankfully, it is usually for some minor disorder; however, as you can imagine, there are times when this can be a dangerous path.

As with physical illnesses, students will seek out advice from their Yoga teacher or Guru on mental issues before looking to certified professionals. Simple and deep depression, all the way to hearing voices and everything in between, the problems were vast and the solutions unorthodox, and often dangerous.

As well, some people asked for advice in personal matters such as love, marriage, and business. They weren't asking as a friend, but as a student. I declined commenting on such matters. What I find truly amazing is that they thought the wise thing was to ask for my counsel.

Lastly, advising someone on spiritual matters. Well, as I said before, Reincarnation and Karma is the great eliminator. It eliminates the afterlife, heaven, hell, salvation, justification, and sanctification. The belief that we are constantly evolving at our own pace and under our own efforts excuses mistakes…better known as Sin.

John 14:6: Jesus saith unto him, I am the way, the truth, and the life: no man cometh unto the Father, but by me. KJV

Chapter Eleven

Who is this Jesus?

In the Yoga world, Jesus Christ is not out of the picture. Of course, it all depends on your understanding of Jesus Christ. Their view is certainly not a Biblical one. It's distorted. He's misinterpreted, misquoted, and misunderstood. Yet, the Yoga world often uses his name, and always to their advantage.

As stated before, most of what passes as information isn't written down. It is tossed around as if fact. Actually, it is a mixture of speculation and myth, the name of Jesus Christ is just that.

Whenever mentioning Jesus, He's mentioned with respect and reverence, always looked up to as an enlightened being. However, He's never referred to as God, the Son of God, the Redeemer, or Savior, and he never died for anyone or their sins. Some even believe He never really died at all, at least not on the cross.

One premise considers the Bible speaking of Jesus' birth and His early life as a child and then a young boy. After that, there is no mention of Him till he appears again in His early thirties, and begins his ministry.

Some in the Yoga world believe those missing years He spent traveling throughout India, visiting and studying under all the great ancient Gurus, learning all about Yoga.

Since Jesus lived so many different lives, over many thousands of reincarnations, he became an Enlightened Being. Once enlightened, He soon surpassed all his teachers, which explains His great powers.

After His enlightenment, He returned to Jerusalem to start His ministry. The fact His actions caused the birth of a religion is that He gathered devotees and followers who in turn misinterpreted and misunderstood his real purpose. And that was to free the world from their miserable existence, and break free of Reincarnation and Karma through His teachings.

His great Yogic powers also explain all the miracles. For an Enlightened Being it's nothing to heal the sick, raise the dead, or walk on water – you can do it, too.

Many also credit his great command of the universe to explain his power over death itself. Able to control his body, he slowed his heart down to give the impression he'd died. Then after three days, his followers took him from his grave, and he went to live and practice in peace far from the crowds. It's even thought by some he married and raised a family.

Hebrews 13:8: Jesus Christ the same yesterday, and today, and forever. KJV

****

Using this new and revised definition of Jesus Christ, His name is mentioned often. Sadly, anyone with an elementary understanding of the Bible would know this to be misleading and wrong. However, the people hearing this rubbish have a poor understanding of Jesus, even the ones claiming to be Christians and reared in the Church, but never studied their Bibles.

Besides their distorted representation of God, Jesus, angels, and the universe, in general, verses of the Bible float into the Yoga vocabulary. Of course, the verses they use are always misinterpreted and taken out of context to support their agenda.

It's not just what's transferred from teacher to student. There isn't a well-known Yogi or Guru worth their salt that doesn't travel the world over giving speeches and seminars, as well as having one or more books for sale.

They can be downright shameless. Just as an example: I heard one speaker use Psalm 46:10 - *Be still, and know that I am God*, saying it endorses the use of Yoga Mediation to find God.

Proverbs 30:5-6: Every word of God is tested; He is a shield to those who take refuge in Him. Do not add to His words Or He will reprove you, and you will be proved a liar. KJV

Matthew 24:23: Then if any man shall say unto you, Lo, here is Christ, or there; believe it not. KJV

Chapter Twelve

Charlatans

This chapter is in no way exclusive to Yoga. Anywhere there are vulnerable people seeking the truth, trying to improve themselves and their lives; there will always be someone trying to exploit them. Still, I included this chapter, because of the unique way charlatans work in the Yoga world.

It wasn't always what they said; although, they could spin a yarn and leave your head spinning, it was the tricks of the trade that worked the best, and I do mean tricks.

One so-called holy man would shake his hand in the air and ash would appear between his fingers. He'd then toss the ashes on the heads of his devotees. This they considered to be a blessing.

He had another one of his tricks not done for the masses, only one-on-one. He'd do his waving of his hand in the air, and then a wood splinter appeared in his palm. He'd offer it to the devotee as a gift, claiming it was a sliver of wood from the cross of Jesus.

Levitation is another common trick, as well as predicting the future, both for individuals and the entire world. Of course, no one is keeping score.

I knew of one male Yoga teacher that lured his women students into his bed, claiming that during sex he was mystically lining up their Chakras. This, of course, gave the Kundalini energy a straight path up the spine and to the crown of the head.

I'm glad to say, and I'm sure you are too; eventfully, they found him out and arrested him, but not after causing years of damage to many women.

Another serpent that showed its head a little more often than you'd imagine was channeling. It always followed the same pattern. The person channeling goes into a trance, and then another being takes control of the person and speaks to the audience, giving advice, predicting, and taking questions.

The entity controlling and speaking through them varied from ancient warriors, sagas, aliens from another planet or another realm, and some from long lost civilizations, including Atlantis. All of them come to help the earth and its beings. All of them with wisdom beyond belief, questioned by none, and with strange, mysterious, and regal names.

A side note: Often the voice they spoke in while channeling had an English accent. A coincidence, I suppose.

When they come out of the trance and the channeled being returns to wherever it came from, the person channeling claims they know nothing of what just occurred.

They put on quite a show, one that most people can easily and laughingly see through, as they do with most charlatans. Still, they never lack a fair amount of followers.

2 Timothy 4:3-4: For the time will come when they will not endure sound doctrine; but after their own lusts shall they heap to themselves teachers, having itching ears... KJV

1 John 4:1: Beloved, believe not every spirit, but try the spirits whether they are of God: because many false prophets are gone out into the world. KJV

Matthew 7:15: Beware of false prophets, which come to you in sheep's clothing, but inwardly they are ravening wolves. KJV

Chapter Thirteen

Power

The Yoga realm clearly teaches and believes that humans have not obtained their full potential. With practice, humans can reach great heights; even, as mentioned before, to becoming gods. Though many don't take it that far, they do believe the potential is great.

With this comes great power, not acquired all at once when you achieve enlightenment, but as you progress you gather more and more power. These powers come in all categories, physical, mental, and spiritual.

I feel a need to say now these powers are real; at least to the extent the Yogi believes them to be. If this is because of trickery, hypnosis, the work of demons, or just the sheer want for them to be true, I really couldn't say. I do know that I've seen and experienced things that I cannot explain.

Meditation and Chanting play a large part of progressing and gathering power. There are meditations to help succeed, or obtain wealth, health, give you intuition, the ability to do impossible feats such as astro trajection, walking through walls and on water. You might be able to read minds, interpret dreams, heal diseases, and a host of other unworldly controls over the body, mind, spirit, and the inward and outward world.

As for me, these were some of my experiences. Again, the reason behind these phenomenon I have no explanation.

There are as many types of mediations as there are Gurus, and I tried as many as possible. Some gave me visions; others allowed me to leave my body and many other phenomenon.

Again, as real as they seemed, that does not make them real. What frightens me most is I'm sure there was no trickery or hypnosis, which leaves me with only one alternative. Unholy influences were at play. Who knows how strong those influences would become, if I hadn't stopped living that life, as the saying goes: There but for the grace of God go I.

Genesis 3:5: For God doth know that in the day ye eat thereof, then your eyes shall be opened, and ye shall be as gods, knowing good and evil. KJV

Chapter Fourteen

Life after the Ashram

Actually, I never left the Ashram. The Ashram left me. A hundred-year-old mansion needs constant repair, which gets to be costly. Insurance was a matter, and there were taxes to be paid. All of it needed paying by a household where only a handful made their living in the outside world. For most of them, their only income was from teaching Yoga. In short, the bills went unpaid, and the Ashram closed.

Having an income other than teaching it was just pocket-change for me, I rented an apartment, went to work each day, and went on with my life. All the while, thinking Yoga would remain a part of my life, but the teaching would end. I was wrong.

The world was so Yoga crazy, and the demand for teachers was great. I got calls from Yoga schools within a fifty mile radius. The city called me wanting classes taught at municipal centers. Large companies wanted classes taught to their employees, as part of their good-health programs. The world was my oyster and Yoga was the pearl.

Many of my old students at the Ashram followed me and began showing up at my classes, as well as taking on new students.

One would think I had it made, but as all things not done for the Lord, there is always a fly in the ointment.

With so many people hanging on my every word, looking for answers, thinking more of me than I did of myself, my ego became the size of all outdoors.

In the words of Max Lagracé - Devolve your ego before it devolves yourself.

John 5:30: I can of mine own self do nothing: as I hear, I judge: and my judgment is just; because I seek not mine own will, but the will of the Father which hath sent me. KJV

Proverbs 16:5: Every one that is proud in heart is an abomination to the LORD: though hand join in hand, he shall not be unpunished. KJV

Chapter Fifteen

Guru

Break down the word Guru into two parts – GU and RU; you have GU that stands for darkness, and RU, light that dispels it. So, together – Guru, we have a symbol for anything that drives out the darkness of ignorance in the devotee. This may include anything from an experience, or a dream, a vision, a feeling, a visitation, a book, just about anything or anyone. However, for this chapter we are only looking at Guru in the form of another human being.

A Guru is a teacher, not just any teacher. He is advanced in the physical and the spiritual with a deep understanding of the universe. Though most Gurus are men, there are many women Gurus. Some are famous, some are not. Some have many devotees, some have only a few. They're considered holy men and women – saints.

Most often, many of the well-known Gurus will only teach a Yoga class to a small group. Lectures take most of their time. Learning, sitting at the foot of the Guru a devotee considers sacred. People come from all over the world to meet the Guru and hear what they have to say. As well, some Gurus may go on tour of different countries. Although, most Gurus are from the East, lately, Gurus have been popping up in the West.

One of the most disturbing aspects about Gurus is the connection between the devotee and Guru. People search long and far, for many years to find their Guru. That's right, not just any Guru, but *their* Guru, the one they're destined to study under, the one that will secure their destiny.

Finding your true Guru is like finding your third and spiritual parent with a connection deeper than you will ever have with anyone. They are your salvation!

How does a holy person become holy? He becomes holy because of much practice through many lifetimes, collecting good Karma, and burning away much of their bad Karma, if having none at all. They're enlightened beings, no longer needing a body of flesh. The only reason they are still in the body and on the earth is to serve. It is their sacrifice for the world, and in time they will leave this mortal coil and enter their final manifestation.

The doctrine of the Guru is overwhelming. They have a say in every facet of your life. They teach on when, where, and how to; sleep, eat, drink, dress, marriage, sex, and so much more; even so far as the positioning of furniture in your home.

If you know what is good for you, you must take everything they say to heart. After all, remember, your salvation is in their hands.

Often, devotees not only lift Gurus on high, but they worship them. They believe just being in the presence will burn away collected bad Karma, and help you to progress in your Yogic journey.

Many devotees hang pictures of their Guru around their home. Some may even make a small altar, on it a photo of their Guru where they will worship, leave flowers and offerings, and burn candles and incense. They also believe that staring into the eyes of the Guru (alive or deceased) in the photo can have a positive affect on the student.

As said before, a Guru can be male or female. Only, that's not where it stops. The Guru can be dead. Prayers and worship of the image of a deceased Guru is just as powerful as one that is alive.

Ecclesiastes 9:5: For the living know that they will die; but the dead know nothing, and they have no more reward, for the memory of them is forgotten. NKJV

Psalm 146:4: His spirit departs, he returns to his earth; In that very day his plans perish. NKJV

There is nothing wrong with seeking out advice or instruction from someone on spiritual matters; however, as the ultimate authority, that's another matter. A Christian has only one authority and that is Jesus Christ.

Matthew 28:18: And Jesus came and spoke to them, saying, "All authority has been given to me in heaven and on earth. NKJV

John 17:2: As thou hast given him power over all flesh, that he should give eternal life to as many as thou hast given him. KJV

John 3:31: He who comes from above is above all; he who is of the earth is earthly and speaks of the earth. He who comes from heaven is above all. NKJV

Chapter Sixteen

Yoga and the West

The West has always had a fascination with the East, and a soft spot for its Yogis. Yoga has silently seeped into the culture of the West.

I know this may sound like a joke, but it isn't.

Two people walk into a casino for the first time in their life. They both gamble. One leaves and goes home. The other stays and continues gambling till they've lost everything.

Two people walk into a bar for the first time. They both have something to drink. One finishes their drink and goes home. The other turns into an alcoholic and his entire life turns to ruin.

It is the same with Yoga. There are thousands of people who take a few classes, and in the end walk away. Yet, there are thousands who start off innocently, and then go further into it, spiraling out of control.

However, as stated before there is no such thing as innocent Yoga. You are playing with fire, a fire that does burn in this life.

The West is slowly coming apart at the seams. The influences of the world are slowly tearing us away from civilization, away from the church, and away from God. All of us know this.

Why is it happening? The answer is in the Bible. The Devil is a lion looking to devour us.

How is it happening? By slowly infiltrating our society with all that is ungodly, and Yoga is a part of that.

We know the old fable:

If you want to cook a frog, and you drop the frog in boiling water, it will jump out and hop away. But if you place the frog in a pot of cold water and place the pot over a slow burning flame, the water will heat so slowly the frog will hardly notice the changes. In time you will have a cooked frog.

That is what is happening, now. Slowly indoctrinated with things that may seem innocent at the beginning, and they just might be. Once we accept it in this mundane form, it slowly changes, showing its true colors. But, by then it's too late. It is part of our lives. And we find it far harder to get out as it was to get in.

This is happening everywhere, and most people are unaware. After all, what harm can there be? It's only stretching, and you can even buy Yoga pants at any convenience store.

2 Thessalonians 3:3: But the Lord is faithful, who will establish you and guard you from the evil one.: NKJV

Chapter Seventeen

Why I left Yoga

Every twelve years, in India, the Hindus hold the festival of Kumbh Mela along the Ganges River for several weeks. Millions of Hindus make the pilgrimage to bathe in the Ganges, celebrate their faith, and converse with Yogis and Gurus from around the country.

Legend has it that a simple farmer decided to attend the festival, traveling hundreds of miles. When he was within a hundred miles of the festival, he came to the bank of a river. It was too deep to wade across and too far to swim; however, there was a rowboat moored along the bank for public use.

Just then, a famous and powerful Guru showed up on the same riverbank.

"Oh, magnificent Guru," said the farmer. "Allow me the honor to row you across to the other side."

"That won't be necessary," replied the Guru. "I have no need for boats. However, you can row yourself across, and I will meet you on the opposite shore."

So, the farmer got into the rowboat, and paddled across the river. Standing on the other riverbank, he looked back to see the Guru still standing on the opposite shore.

The Guru blinked his eyes, disappeared, and in the next instant reappeared on the opposite shore, standing next to the farmer.

"Oh, great Guru, you truly are a powerful Yogi. Tell me, how does a person gain such power?"

The Guru replied with pride, "It took me twenty years of Yogic practice to be able to achieve the feat you've just witnessed."

The farmer smiled. "I rowed across this river. It took ten minutes for me to cross. You, on the other hand, have taken twenty years."

****

That is what Yoga became for me, much effort for uselessness. The hype blinded me. The spiritual hunger that pressed me on was now the force that made me quit, as I realized it was just a dead end, leaving me empty.

It was the old phrase – All that glitters is not gold.

Thankfully, that spiritual hunger continued to gnaw at me, pressing me on. I began checking out different religions, visiting churches, temples, and masques, going to lectures, and reading everything I could get me hands on. Only, now, I armed myself with a new skepticism that made me question everything. And everything came up short, until I took a new and deeper look at Christianity.

My skepticism ferreted out flaws in every belief system, but never in Christianity or the Bible. Then I realized why. Christianity is not a system at all. And if you find fault in it, it is because you're misinformed or you misunderstood. I can identify with that.

From a child to an adult, I'd tried reading the Bible, and it made little sense to me, it always came up short. Actually, it was I that came up short. For without the Holy Spirit the Bible is just another book.

It is contrary to all logic. Logic says, "I'll believe it, when I see it.", where as with Christianity, "I'll see it, when I believe it."

When you give your life to Christ and the Holy Spirit enters you, all the pieces fall into place. Now, I had an interpreter helping me, doing what I couldn't do on my own.

Once reborn and reading the Bible, it didn't take long to see how much Yoga contradicts the word of God.

2 Corinthians 5:17: Therefore if any man be in Christ, he is a new creature: old things are passed away. Behold, all things are become new. KJV

Chapter Eighteen

Conclusion

So, in conclusion, we have many aspects to recount, all of them important.

First and most important, and I know many people do not want to believe this and they will argue till they're blue in the face, there is no innocent Yoga.

Even if all you do is the physical exercises and none of the Meditation, Mantras, or Chants, the exercises are intended to stir up forces that are not in your control and if not demonic are definitely not Biblical.

There is nothing wrong with stretching exercises. Join an aerobics class, but there is no way a Christian can safely practice any part of Yoga.

This brings us to the next point. There in no Christian friendly Yoga. Repeating the name of God over and over as a Mantra doesn't make it right, rehashing over and over a Bible verse as a Chant is wrong. None of these twists and turns can ever make it acceptable. If it walks like a duck, and quacks like a duck...well, you know the rest.

For the Holy Spirit to dwell within us, we must empty ourselves with Humility and Gratitude.

But to empty yourself, thoughtless, without direction, leaves you open to anything. And know that if there is any unprotected space, an unnatural demonic force will surely take advantage of the situation. Like any parasite, it will find a home, and nestle in, living off the host.

The word of God is infallible; the word of man, even from someone well-meaning is no substitute.

Any power you or anyone else possesses is from God, and there is nothing you can do to get it.

The first lie was from the Devil. It is also the greatest, the most dangerous, and the most damaging. You are not God and you will never be.

Don't start, and if you have, stop; it is never too late.

Isaiah 1:18: Come now, and let us reason together, saith the LORD: though your sins be as scarlet, they shall be as white as snow; though they be red like crimson, they shall be as wool. KJV

THE END

For more information or to order this book (single or bulk copies)
contact the publisher at info@advbooks.com

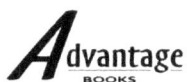

*A*dvantage
BOOKS

advbookstore.com

www.ingramcontent.com/pod-product-compliance
Lightning Source LLC
Chambersburg PA
CBHW072039060426
42449CB00010BA/2359